INTRODUCTION

Obesity is a major public health problem, affecting millions of people worldwide. The conventional wisdom is that obesity is caused by a calorie surplus, but Dr. Melissa argues that this is not the whole story. In his book, The Obesity Protocol, Dr. Melissa explains that obesity is caused by insulin resistance, a condition in which the body's cells become resistant to the hormone insulin. Insulin is responsible for transporting glucose (sugar) from the bloodstream into the cells, where it can be used for energy.

When cells become resistant to insulin, glucose builds up in the bloodstream, leading to weight gain.

Dr. Melissa also argues that intermittent fasting is the best way to lose weight and reverse insulin resistance.

Intermittent fasting is an eating pattern that alternates between eating and fasting intervals. Intermittent fasting can be done in a variety of ways, but the most popular is to fast for 16 hours and then eat within an 8-hour window.

In The Obesity Protocol, Dr. Melissa provides a comprehensive overview of the science of obesity and weight loss. He also shares his own story of weight loss and health improvement through intermittent fasting.

The book is a must-read for anyone who is struggling with obesity or who wants to learn more about the science of weight loss.

Genetics Because of their DNA, some people are more inclined to be obese than others.

Environment: The environment in which we live can make it difficult to maintain a healthy weight. For example, many people have access to unhealthy foods and lack access to healthy foods.

Behavioral factors: Our behaviors, such as our eating habits and physical activity levels, can also contribute to obesity.

The obesity epidemic is a serious problem, but there are things that we can do to address it. We can make changes to our environment to make it easier to make healthy choices.

We can also change our behaviors, such as eating healthier foods and getting more physical activity

The obesity epidemic is a challenge, but it is one that we can overcome. By working together, we can create a healthier future for ourselves and our children.

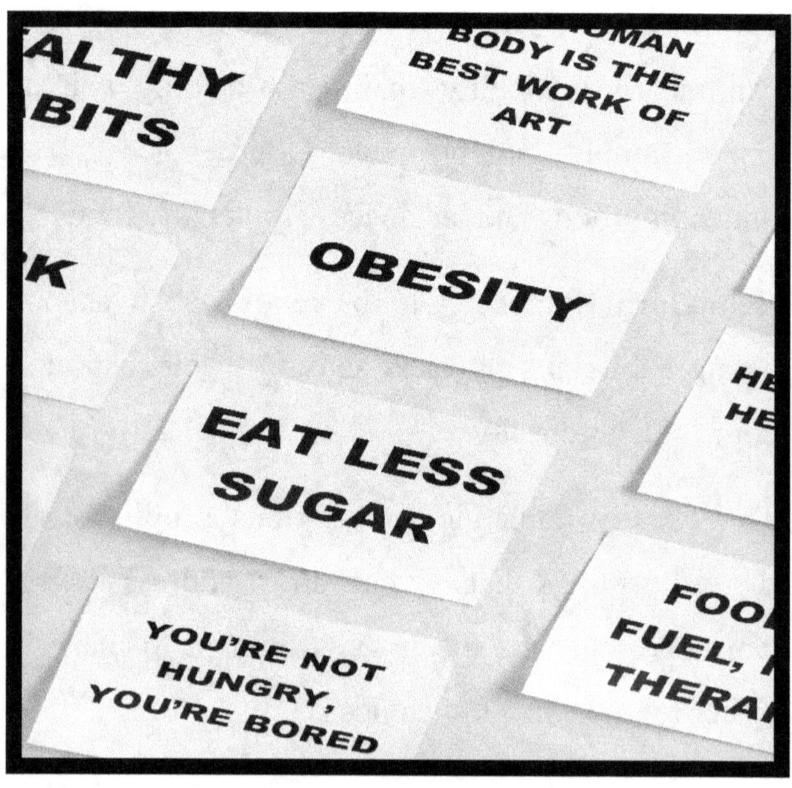

Make healthy foods more affordable and accessible.

Create more opportunities for physical activity.

Educate individuals on the dangers of obesity and how to avoid it.

Support research into new treatments for obesity.

By taking these steps, we can make a difference in the fight against the obesity epidemic. We can create a healthier future for ourselves and our children

THE FAILURE OF DIETS

Obesity is a huge public health issue that affects millions of individuals around the world.

Most people who lose weight on a diet will regain it within a year.

There are several reasons why diets fail, but one of the biggest reasons is that they are not sustainable.

Most diets are too restrictive and difficult to follow. They require people to give up their favorite foods and eat foods that they don't enjoy. This makes it very difficult to stick to the diet in the long term.

Another reason why diets fail is that they don't address the underlying causes of obesity.

Obesity is a complex problem that is caused by a combination of factors, including genetics, environment, and behavior.

Diets that focus only on food and exercise are not going to be effective in the long term.

The Obesity Code is a book that challenges the conventional wisdom about weight loss. Dr. Melissa D. Johnson argues that the key to losing weight is not to eat less and exercise more, but to control insulin levels.

Insulin is a hormone that the pancreas produces. It aids the body's ability to store glucose, or blood sugar, in cells. The body stores fat when insulin levels are high. The body burns fat when insulin levels are low.

Dr. Melissa believes that the current obesity epidemic is caused by a high-carb diet that leads to high insulin levels.

These high insulin levels cause the body to store fat and make it difficult to lose weight.

The Obesity Protocol offers a new approach to weight loss that is based on controlling insulin levels.

Dr. Melissa recommends eating a low-carb diet that is high in fat and moderate in protein. This diet will help to keep insulin levels low, which will allow the body to burn fat and lose weight.

The Obesity Protocol is a controversial book, but it has a lot of evidence to support its claims.

Dr. Melissa has been studying the effects of diet and insulin levels for over 20 years, and he has helped thousands of people lose weight and keep it off.

If you are struggling with obesity, I encourage you to read This Obesity Code. It may just change your life.

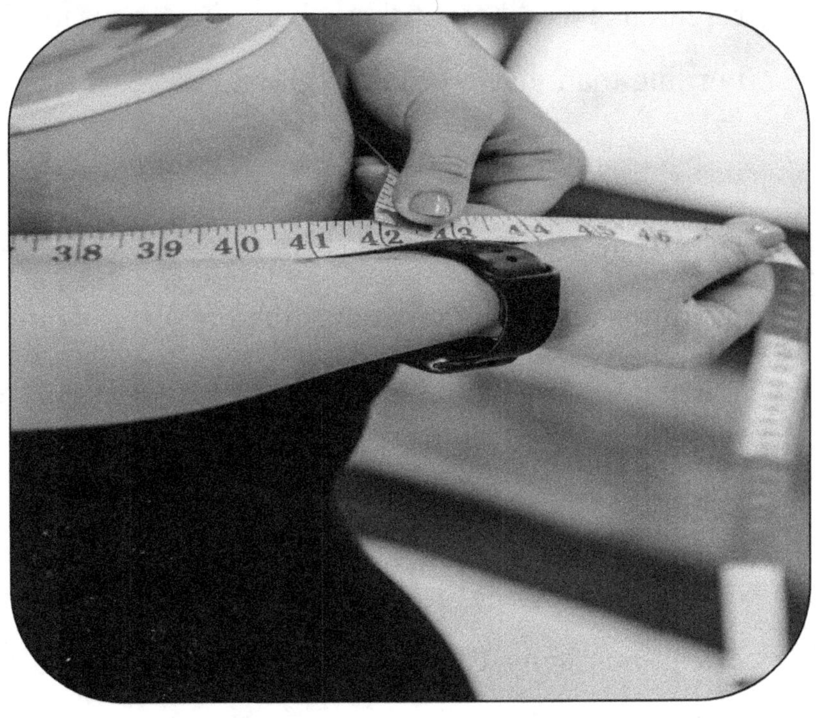

THE NEW SCIENCE OF FAT BURNING

The traditional view of fat burning is that it is a simple matter of calories in vs. calories out In other words, you will lose weight if you expend more calories than you ingest. However, recent research has shown that there is more to fat burning than just calories.

One of the key factors in fat burning is insulin. Insulin is a hormone that aids the body's utilization of glucose for energy. When we eat a meal, our blood sugar levels rise and insulin is released to help the cells take up glucose.

However, if we eat too many carbohydrates or too often, our cells can become resistant to insulin.

This means that they don't take up glucose as efficiently, and the excess glucose is stored as fat.

Another important factor in fat burning is the body's metabolism. The rate at which the body burns calories is referred to as metabolism. Several things can affect metabolism, including age, genetics, and activity level.

Finally, the body's ability to burn fat is also affected by the type of exercise we do. Exercise that is high-intensity and short-duration, such as interval training, is more effective for fat burning than exercise that is low-intensity and long-duration, such as steady-state cardio.

The new science of fat burning is still evolving, but we are learning more about how to target fat cells and burn fat more effectively.

15 [Dr. Melissa D. Johnson]

Intermittent fasting: Intermittent fasting is an eating habit that alternates between periods of eating and fasting. There are many different ways to do intermittent fasting, but the most common is to fast for 16 hours and eat during an 8-hour window.

Low-carb diet: A low-carb diet restricts carbohydrate intake. This can help to improve insulin sensitivity and make it easier to burn fat.

High-protein diet: A high-protein diet is a diet that emphasizes protein intake.

Protein can help to boost metabolism and prevent muscle loss during weight loss.

<u>**Exercise:**</u> Exercise is an essential component of any weight loss program. Exercise can help to burn calories, improve insulin sensitivity, and build muscle.

<u>**Supplements:**</u> Several supplements may be helpful for fat-burning, such as green tea extract, caffeine, and conjugated linoleic acid (CLA).

<u>**It is important to note that there is no one-size-fits-all approach to fat burning.**</u> What works for one person might not work for the next. It is important to find a strategy that is sustainable and that you can stick with in the long term.

CHAPTER 1

The Hormonal Code is a term coined by Dr. Melissa D. Johnson in his book The Obesity Protocol. It refers to the idea that obesity is caused by hormonal imbalances, specifically insulin resistance. Insulin is a hormone that helps the body use glucose for energy.

When we eat a meal, our blood sugar levels rise and insulin is released to help the cells take up glucose. However, if we eat too many carbohydrates or too often, our cells can become resistant to insulin.

This means that they don't take up glucose as efficiently, and the excess glucose is stored as fat.

The Hormonal Code suggests that obesity is not caused by a calorie surplus but by insulin resistance. This is because when we are insulin resistant, our bodies are constantly producing insulin in an attempt to get the cells to take up glucose. This high level of insulin can lead to weight gain, even if we are not eating a lot of calories.

The Hormonal Code also suggests that the best way to lose weight and reverse insulin resistance is to intermittent fasting. Intermittent fasting is an eating pattern that alternates between eating and fasting intervals. There are many different ways to do intermittent fasting, but the most common is to fast for 16 hours and eat during an 8-hour window.

Intermittent fasting is effective for weight loss and improving insulin sensitivity.

It can also help to improve other health markers, such as blood pressure, cholesterol, and blood sugar levels.

In addition to intermittent fasting, Dr. Melissa D. Johnson also recommends making other lifestyle changes, such as eating a low-carb diet and getting regular exercise. These changes can help to improve insulin sensitivity and make it easier to lose weight and keep it off.

THE KEY HORMONES INVOLVED IN FAT-BURNING AND WEIGHT LOSS:

<u>Insulin:</u> Insulin is a hormone that aids the body's utilization of glucose for energy. When we eat a meal, our blood sugar levels rise and insulin is released to help the cells take up glucose. However, if we eat too many carbohydrates or too often, our cells can become resistant to insulin. This means that they don't take up glucose as efficiently, and the excess glucose is stored as fat.

<u>Ghrelin:</u> When our stomach is empty, it is released. It is released when our stomach is empty.

<u>Leptin:</u> Leptin is a hormone that causes us to feel satiated. It is released by fat cells.

<u>**Thyroid hormones:**</u> Thyroid hormones aid in metabolism regulation.

<u>**Cortisol:**</u> Cortisol is a stress hormone that can promote weight gain.

The Hormonal Code is a complex concept, but it is an important one to understand if you are struggling with obesity.

By understanding the role of hormones in weight loss, you can make better choices about your diet and lifestyle and improve your chances of success.

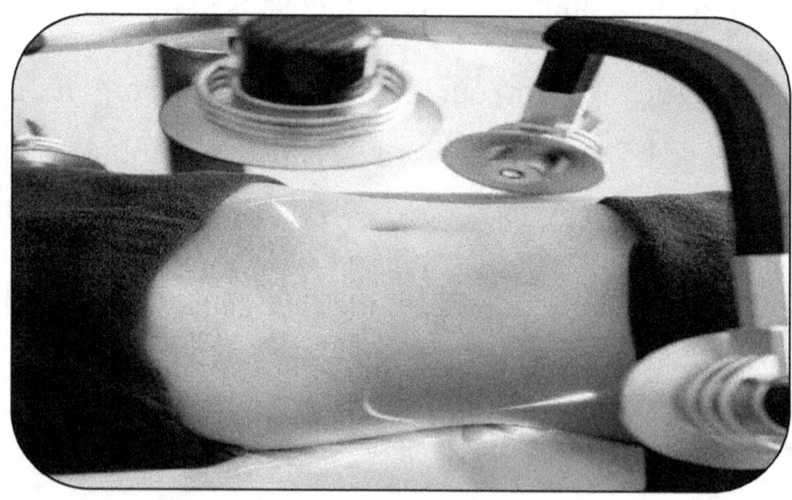

THE HORMONAL DANCE OF OBESITY

The hormonal dance of obesity is a complex interplay of hormones that can lead to weight gain and obesity. When the body is in a state of insulin resistance, the pancreas produces more and more insulin to try to keep blood sugar levels under control. This high level of insulin can lead to fat storage and weight gain.

Insulin resistance is often caused by a diet that is high in refined carbohydrates and sugar.

These foods cause a rapid rise in blood sugar levels, which triggers the release of insulin. Over time, the body becomes less sensitive to insulin, and more insulin is needed to keep blood sugar levels under control.

In addition to insulin, other hormones are also involved in the hormonal dance of obesity.

Leptin is a hormone that fat cells manufacture. It tells the brain when the body has enough fat stored. When leptin levels are high, the brain tells the body to stop eating. However, in obese people, leptin levels are often low, which can lead to overeating.

Ghrelin is another hormone that is involved in the hormonal dance of obesity. Ghrelin is produced by the stomach and it tells the brain when it is time to eat. In obese people, ghrelin levels are often high, which can lead to overeating.

The hormonal dance of obesity is a complex and ever-changing process. However, by understanding how these hormones work, we can better understand the causes of obesity and develop more effective treatments.

<u>Here are some tips for managing the hormonal dance of obesity:</u>

Eat a diet that is low in refined carbohydrates and sugar.

Get regular exercise.

Get enough sleep.

Manage stress.

By following these tips, you can help to keep your hormones in balance and reduce your risk of obesity.

CHAPTER 2

Insulin resistance is a condition in which the cells of the body become less receptive to the hormone insulin. This means that insulin is less effective at transporting glucose, or blood sugar, into the cells. As a result, blood sugar levels can rise to unhealthy levels.

Insulin resistance is a major risk factor for type 2 diabetes, heart disease, and other chronic diseases. It is estimated that over 80% of people with type 2 diabetes are insulin resistant.

<u>Genetics:</u> Some people are more likely to develop insulin resistance due to their genes.

<u>Obesity:</u> Excess body fat, especially around the waist, can increase insulin resistance.

<u>Physical inactivity:</u> Lack of exercise can also contribute to insulin resistance.

<u>Poor diet:</u> A diet high in refined carbohydrates and sugar can increase insulin resistance.

<u>Stress:</u> Stress can also lead to insulin resistance.

If you are insulin resistant, there are several things you can do to improve your insulin sensitivity and reduce your risk of Type 2 diabetes and other chronic diseases are on the rise.

These include:

Losing weight: Losing weight, especially around the waist, can help to improve insulin sensitivity.

Getting regular exercise: Exercise can help to improve insulin sensitivity and reduce blood sugar levels.

Eating a healthy diet: A diet that is low in refined carbohydrates and sugar and high in whole grains, fruits, vegetables, and lean protein can help to improve insulin sensitivity.

Managing stress: Stress can lead to insulin resistance, so it is important to find healthy ways to manage stress.

If you are concerned that you may be insulin resistant, talk to your doctor.

Your doctor can perform a blood test to check your insulin levels and blood sugar levels. If you are insulin resistant, your doctor can work with you to develop a treatment plan that will help you improve your insulin sensitivity and reduce your risk of developing type 2 diabetes and other chronic diseases.

Here are some additional tips for improving insulin sensitivity:

Get enough sleep. Sleep deprivation has been linked to insulin resistance in studies.

Avoid sugary drinks. Sugary drinks are a major source of empty calories and can contribute to insulin resistance.

Eat plenty of fiber. Fiber can help to slow down the absorption of glucose into the bloodstream, which can help to improve insulin sensitivity.

Take a probiotic. Probiotics are living microorganisms that aid in digestion and intestinal health. Some studies have shown that probiotics can also help to improve insulin sensitivity.

By following these tips, you can help to improve your insulin sensitivity and reduce your risk of developing type 2 diabetes and other chronic diseases.

CHAPTER 3

THE FASTING CODE

Fasting is one of the most powerful tools we have for improving our health and well-being. It has been shown to reduce inflammation, improve insulin sensitivity, and promote weight loss. In this chapter, we will explore the science of fasting and how it can help you to achieve your health goals.

What is fasting?

Fasting is the act of abstaining from food for some time. Intermittent fasting is the most common type of fasting. Intermittent fasting entails alternating between times of eating and fasting. The most popular intermittent fasting schedule is the 16:8 diet, which involves fasting for 16 hours and eating for 8 hours.

When you eat, your body breaks down the food into glucose, which is used for energy. Insulin is a hormone that aids in the transport of glucose into cells. When you fast, your insulin levels go down and your body starts to burn stored fat for energy.

This process is called **ketosis**. Ketosis is a state in which your body uses ketones for fuel instead of glucose. When fat is broken down, the liver produces ketones.

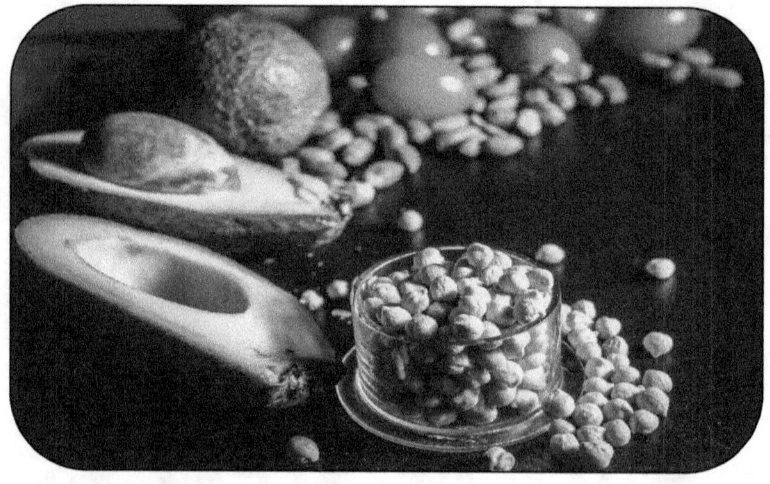

- *Weight loss*

- *Reduced inflammation*

- *Improved insulin sensitivity*

- *Lowered blood pressure*

- *Reduced risk of heart disease*

- *Improved brain function*

- *Increased longevity*

- *How to fast safely*

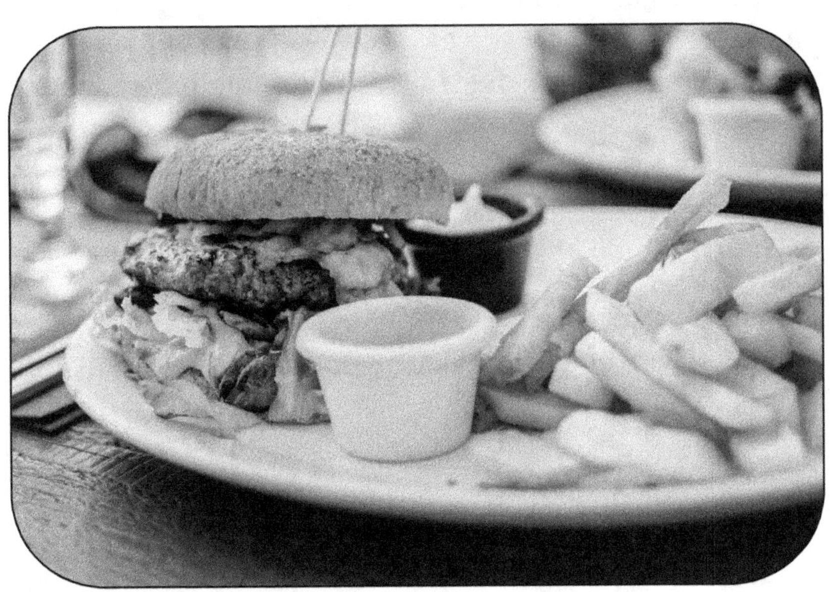

THE DIFFERENT TYPES OF FASTS

THERE ARE TYPES OF FASTS, BUT THE MOST COMMON ARE:

Intermittent fasting: Intermittent fasting entails alternating between times of eating and fasting. The most popular intermittent fasting schedule is the 16:8 diet, which involves fasting for 16 hours and eating for 8 hours.

Alternate-day fasting: Alternate-day fasting involves fasting for one day and eating normally the next day.

5:2 fasting: The 5:2 diet involves fasting for two days per week and eating normally for the other five days.

Long-term fasts: Long-term fasts involve fasting for days or weeks.

The type of fast that is right for you will depend on your individual needs and preferences. If you are new to fasting, it is a good idea to start with a short fast, such as 12 hours or 16 hours. As you get more comfortable with fasting, you can gradually increase the length of your fasts.

It is important to listen to your body and stop fasting if you feel lightheaded or dizzy.

If you have any health conditions, talk to your doctor before starting to fast.

CHAPTER 4

The ketogenic diet is a high-fat, low-carb diet that has been shown to have several health benefits, including weight loss, reduced inflammation, and improved blood sugar control. In this article, we will explore the science behind the ketogenic diet and how it can help you achieve your health goals.

What is the ketogenic diet?

The ketogenic diet is a high-fat, low-carb diet that forces the body to use fat for fuel. When you eat a ketogenic diet, your body breaks down fat into ketones, which are molecules that can be used for energy.

Ketones are produced in the liver when there is not enough glucose available from carbohydrates.

The ketogenic diet is different from other low-carb diets in that it is very restrictive in carbohydrates. Most low-carb diets allow for some carbs, but the ketogenic diet limits carbs to 50 grams or less per day.

This low-carb intake causes the body to enter ketosis, a state in which the body burns fat for fuel.

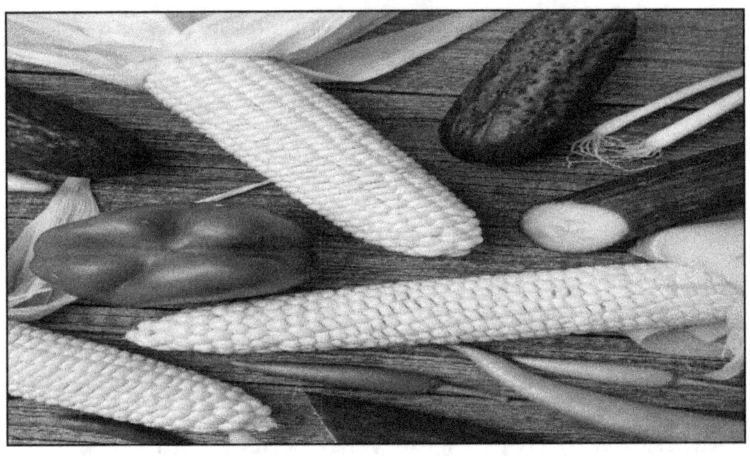

 [Dr. Melissa D. Johnson]

The ketogenic diet has been found to offer various health benefits, including:

Weight loss: The ketogenic diet is a very effective strategy to lose weight. Studies have shown that people who follow a ketogenic diet lose more weight than people who follow other diets.

Reduced inflammation: The ketogenic diet has been shown to reduce inflammation, which is a major risk factor for several diseases, including heart disease, cancer, and diabetes.

Improved blood sugar control: The ketogenic diet has been demonstrated to enhance blood sugar management in persons with type 2 diabetes.

<u>**Improved brain function:**</u> The ketogenic diet has been shown to improve brain function in people with Alzheimer's disease and other neurological disorders.

<u>**Increased energy:**</u> The ketogenic diet can provide a boost of energy, especially in people who are overweight or obese.

Happy healthy life matters a lot

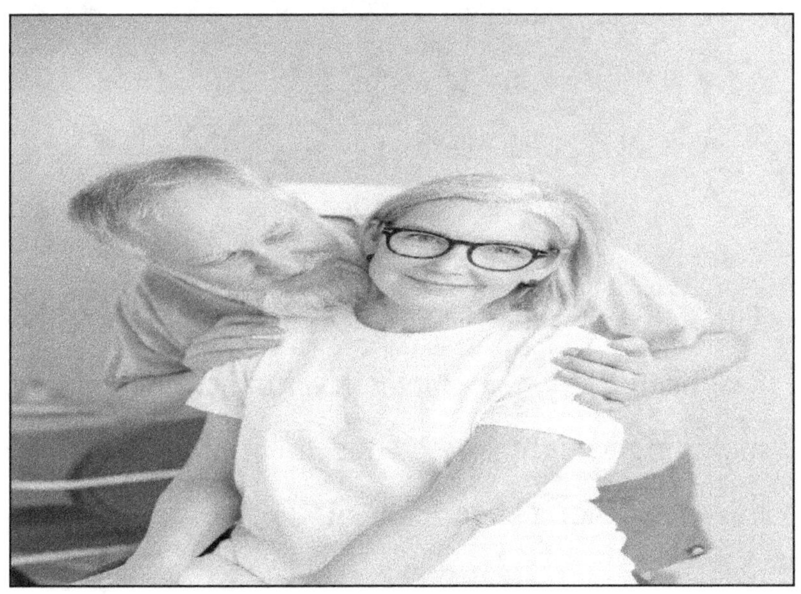

- Eat plenty of healthy fats, such as avocados, olive oil, nuts, and seeds.
- Limit your intake of carbs to 50 grams or less per day.
- Avoid processed foods, sugary drinks, and sugary snacks.
- Drink plenty of water.
- Get regular exercise.

The ketogenic diet is a high-fat, low-carb diet that has been shown to have several health benefits, including weight loss, reduced inflammation, and improved blood sugar control.

CHAPTER 5

In this chapter, we will discuss the lifestyle code that I recommend for people who are trying to lose weight and improve their health. This code is based on the latest scientific research and is designed to help you achieve your weight loss and health goals sustainably.

The lifestyle code is based on the following principles:

- *Eat a healthy diet.*
- *Get regular exercise.*
- *Get enough sleep.*
- *Manage stress.*
- *Find a support system.*

- *Let's take a closer look at each of these ideas.*
- *Eat a healthy diet*

A healthy diet is low in processed foods and high in whole foods. Whole foods are foods that have not been processed or refined. Examples of whole foods include fruits, vegetables, nuts, seeds, and lean protein.

A healthy diet is important for weight loss because it helps to keep your blood sugar levels stable. When your blood sugar levels are stable, you are less likely to feel hungry and overeat.

A healthy diet is also important for overall health because it provides your body with the nutrients it needs to function properly.

Get regular exercise

Exercise is another important part of the lifestyle code. Exercise helps to burn calories and build muscle. Muscle burns more calories than fat, so having more muscle can help you to lose weight and keep it off. Exercise also helps to improve your insulin sensitivity, which is important for preventing type 2 diabetes and other chronic diseases.

Get enough sleep

When you don't get enough sleep, your body creates more of the stress hormone cortisol. Cortisol can contribute to weight gain and other health concerns. Getting enough sleep is vital for keeping a healthy weight and general health.

Manage stress

Stress can also lead to weight gain. When you are stressed, your body creates more of the stress hormone cortisol. Cortisol can contribute to increased appetite and cravings for harmful meals. Managing stress is important for maintaining a healthy weight and overall health.

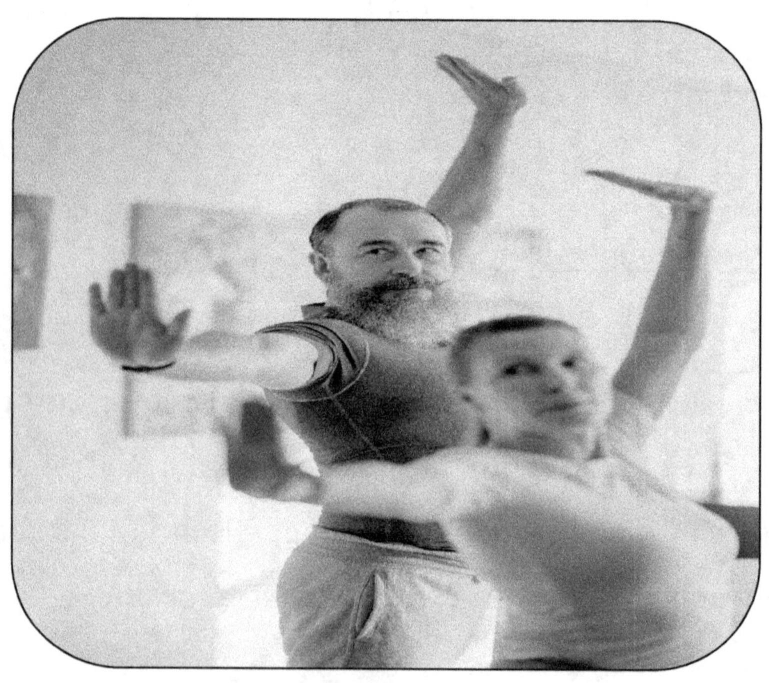

REVERSING OBESITY

Obesity is a serious public health problem that affects millions of people around the world. Obesity is described as having a body mass index (BMI) of 30 or greater. BMI is a measure of body fat based on your height and weight.

Obesity is a risk factor for several chronic diseases, including heart disease, stroke, type 2 diabetes, and some types of cancer.

It can also lead to other health problems, such as sleep apnea, joint pain, and depression.

<u>Eating a healthy diet.</u> A healthy diet is low in saturated fat, trans fat, cholesterol, and sodium. It is also high in fruits, vegetables, and whole grains.

<u>Getting regular exercise.</u> Exercise helps to burn calories and build muscle. Muscle burns more calories than fat, so having more muscle can help you to lose weight and keep it off.

<u>Finding a support system.</u> Having a support system can help you to stay on track with your weight loss goals. This could include friends, family, or a support group.

If you are struggling to lose weight on your own, you may want to talk to your doctor about obesity treatment options. There are several medications and surgical procedures that can help you to lose weight and keep it off.

Reversal of obesity is a lifelong process. It takes time, effort, and commitment. But it is possible to achieve. By following the tips above, you can improve your health and reduce your risk of chronic diseases.

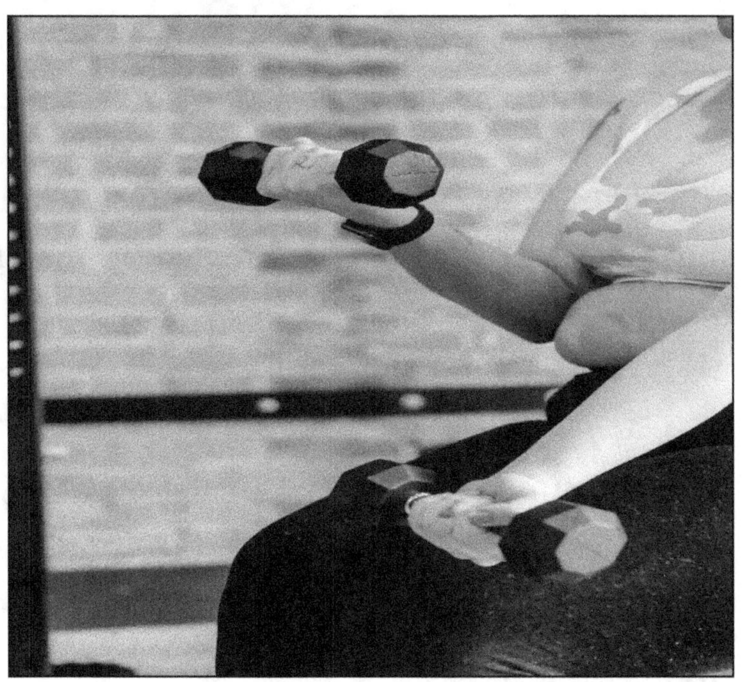

<u>Set realistic goals.</u> Don't try to lose too much weight too quickly. Aim to lose 1-2 pounds per week.

<u>Make small changes to your diet and lifestyle.</u> Don't try to change everything all at once.

Start by making one or two small changes, and then gradually add more changes as you are able.

<u>Find an exercise routine that you enjoy and that you can stick with.</u> Exercise should be fun and something that you look forward to doing.

<u>Be patient.</u> It takes time to lose weight and keep it off. Don't get disheartened if you don't see results quickly. Just stay at it and you will eventually attain your goals.

CONCLUSION

In this book, Dr. Melissa has presented a compelling case for the role of insulin resistance in the development of obesity and other chronic diseases. She has also outlined several strategies for reversing insulin resistance and losing weight, including intermittent fasting, low-carb diets, and exercise.

Believe that (This bookwork is an important contribution to the field of obesity research)

She has helped to shed light on the complex relationship between insulin and weight gain, and she has offered several practical strategies for people who are struggling with obesity.

I highly recommend this book to anyone interested in learning more about the science of obesity and its treatment. It is a well-written and informative book that will challenge your current understanding of weight loss.

The Future of Weight Loss

The future of weight loss is bright. We are learning more and more about the science of obesity, and we are developing new and effective treatments. With the right information and support, people can overcome obesity and enjoy a healthy, happy life.

<u>**Here are some of the things that I believe will be important for the future of weight loss:**</u>

- *More research into the causes of obesity. We need to understand more about why people become obese to develop more effective treatments.*

- *More development of new treatments for obesity. There are several promising new treatments for obesity, such as bariatric surgery and new medications. These treatments need to be further developed and tested so that they can be made available to more people.*

- *More public awareness of obesity. Obesity is a serious public health problem, and we need to do a better job of educating the public about its causes and consequences.*

- *More support for people who are trying to lose weight. People who are trying to lose weight need support from their family, friends, and healthcare providers.*